Letters
to my heart

Diary

Free Life ✶ Compass

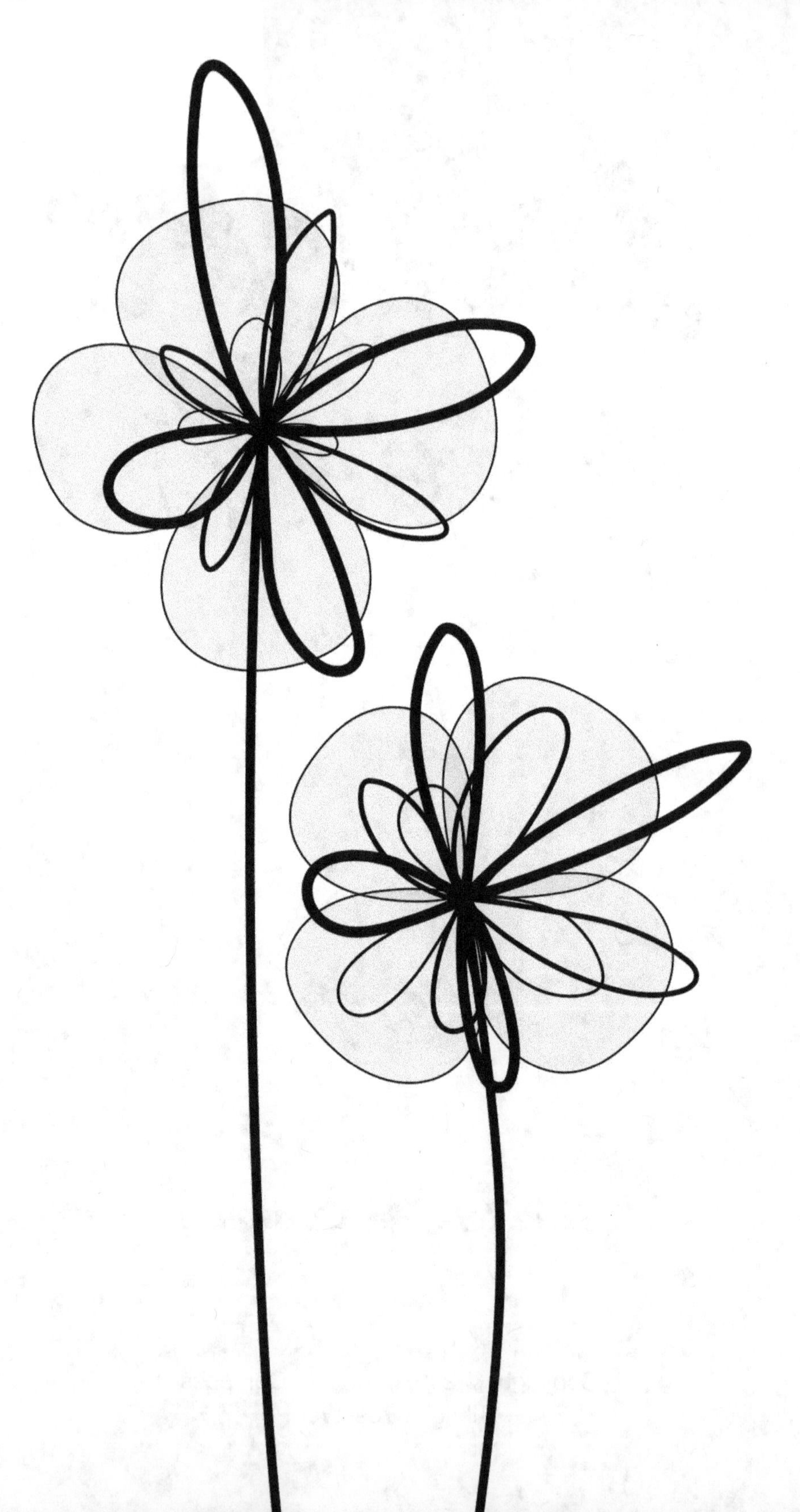

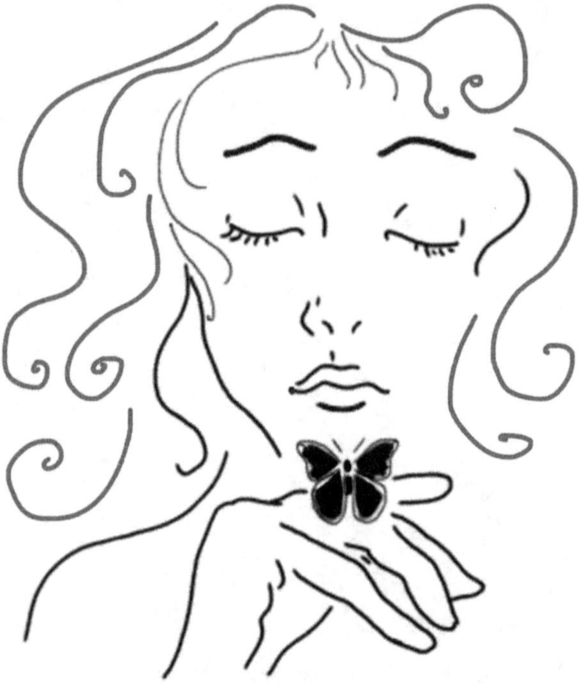

Keep love in your heart.
A life without it
is like a sunless
garden when
the flowers are dead.

Oscar Wilde

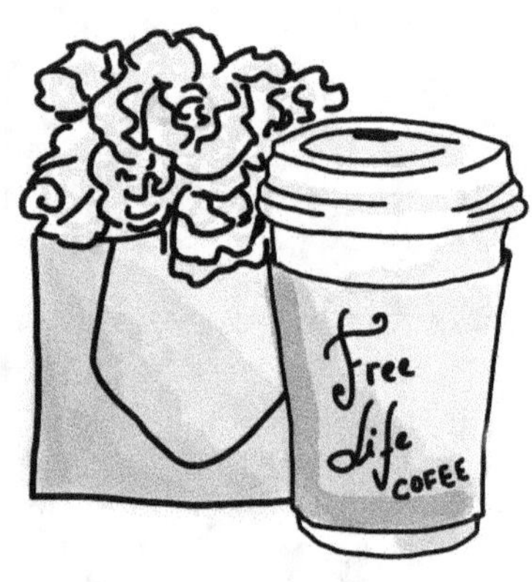

"The primary cause of
unhappiness is never
the situation, but your
thoughts about it.
Be aware of the thoughts
you are thinking."

Eckhart Tolle

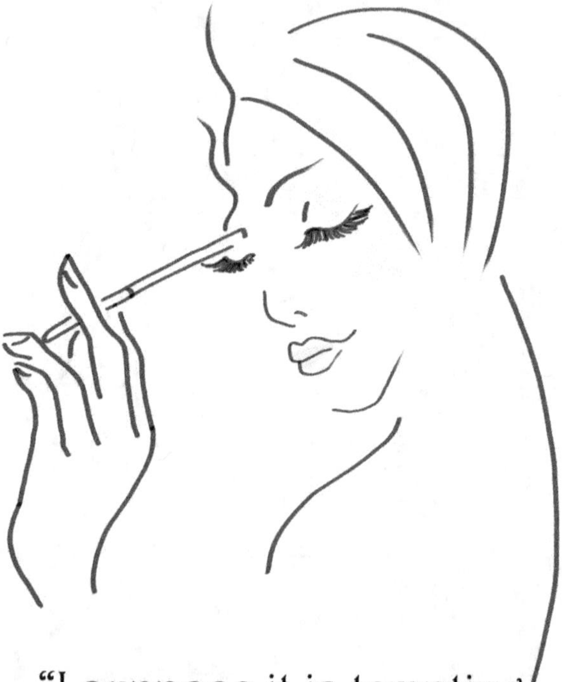

"I suppose it is tempting,
if the only tool you have
is a hammer, to treat
everything as if
it were a nail."

Abraham H. Maslow

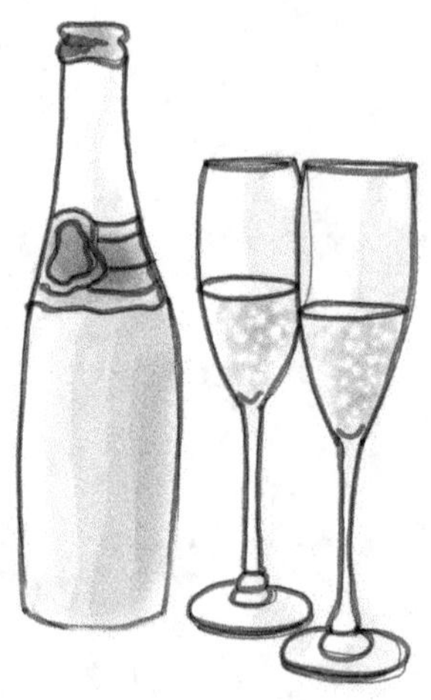

"A wonderful fact
to reflect upon,
that every human creature
is constituted to be that
profound secret
and mystery to every other."

Charles Dickens

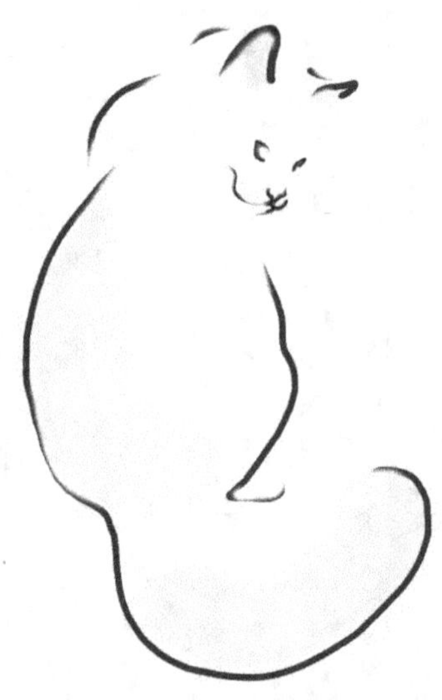

"According to
Madam Pomfrey,
thoughts could
leave deeper scars
than almost anything else."

J.K. Rowling

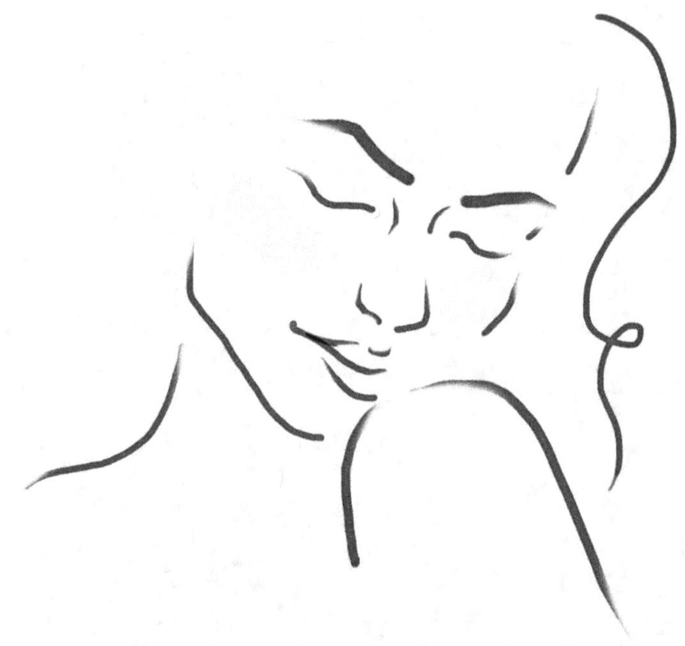

"Our wounds are
often the openings
into the best and most
beautiful part of us."

David Richo

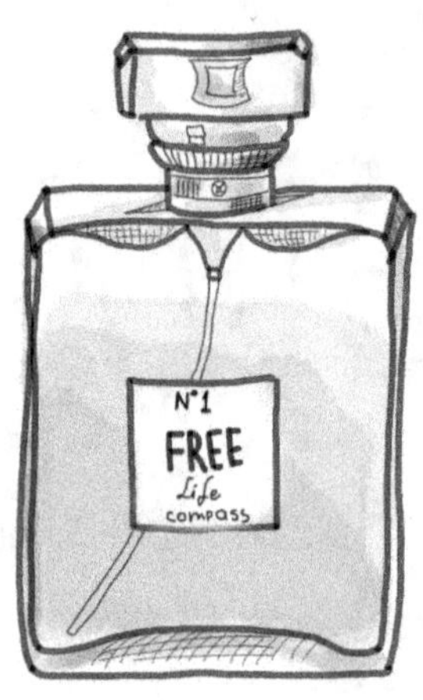

"People often say that this or that
person has not yet found himself.
But the self is not something
one finds, it is something
one creates."

Thomas Szasz

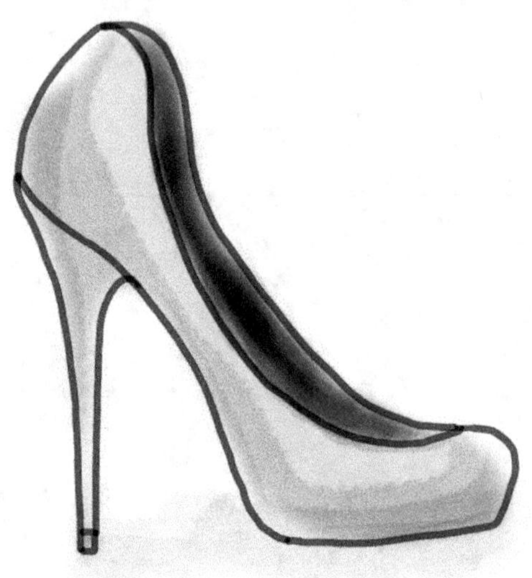

A man wrapped up in
himself makes
a very small parcel.

John Ruskin

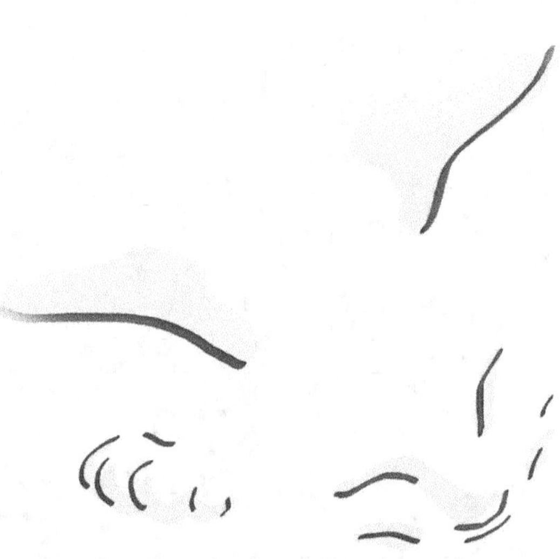

"When the heart speaks,
the mind finds it
indecent to object."

Milan Kundera

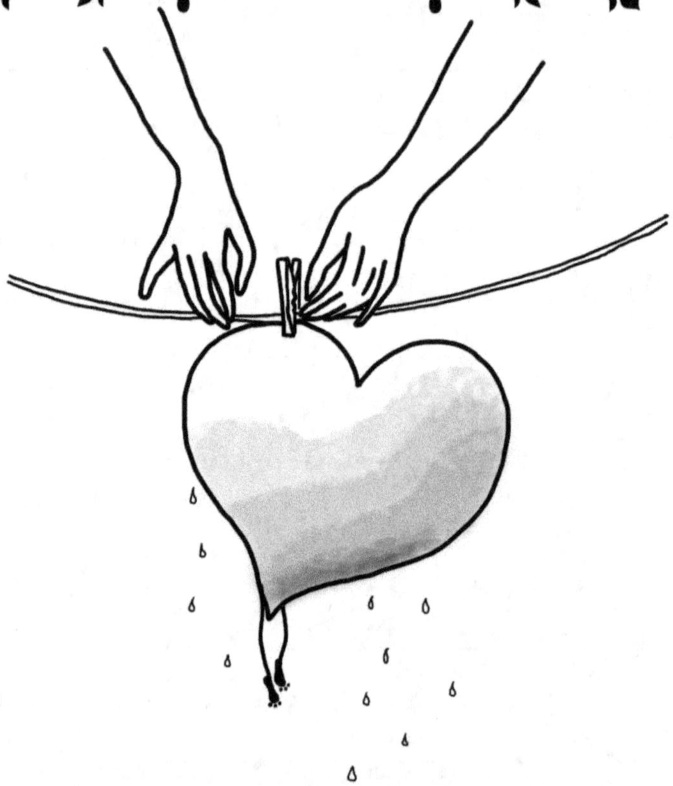

"To find out what is truly
individual in ourselves,
profound reflection is needed;
and suddenly we realize how
uncommonly difficult the
discovery of individuality is."

C.G. Jung

You'll never find
peace of mind
until you listen
to your heart.

George Michael

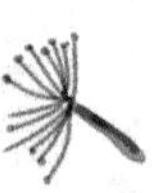

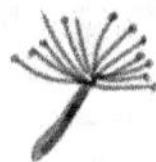

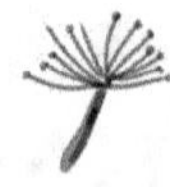

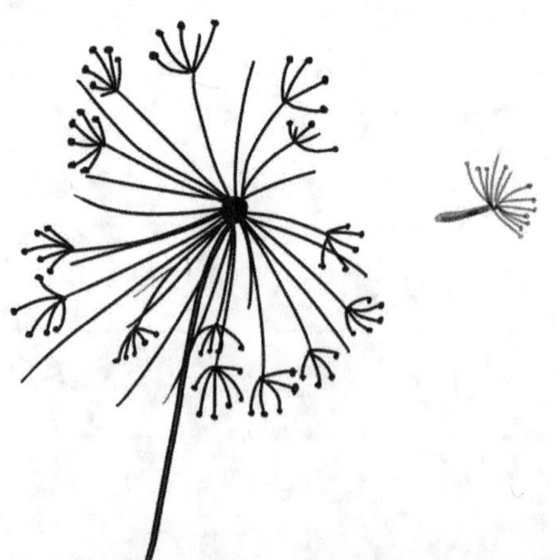